D0627850

FASTING

Father Slavko Barbarić, O.F.M.

FASTING

Franciscan University Press
Franciscan University of Steubenville
Steubenville, Ohio 43952

© 1988 Franciscan University Press
All Rights Reserved

Cover Design: Art Mancuso

Published by:
  Franciscan University Press
  Franciscan University of Steubenville
  Steubenville, Ohio 43952

Printed in the United States of America

ISBN: 0-940535-12-2

REFLECTIONS

The elderly woman, Anna, worshiped night and day, fasting and praying (Lk 2:37). Jesus fasted: "After fasting forty days and nights, he was hungry" (Mt 4:2). Scripture contains many references to fasting, a practice which has been lost in the modern day Church. The scriptural concept of fasting is often misunderstood and therefore, not seen in its proper role in the spiritual life.

The word **fasting** comes from a Hebrew word which literally means "to cover or shut one's mouth." The Greek word means "not to eat." Strictly speaking, fasting is a voluntary abstinence from food, not as an end in itself, but as a means to holiness. Practically speaking, fasting goes beyond the realm of food into our actions and thoughts.

In one of the early messages at Medugorje, the Virgin Mary reportedly said that we have forgotten the value of fasting. She reminded us that wars and natural catastrophies can be averted by prayer and fasting. •The Virgin said that many people have substituted almsgiving for fasting. By excluding fasting from our daily life, we are excluding an important element in growing in holiness which cannot be gained otherwise.

We are all called to fast, even the elderly, the sick, and the young. However, not all are called to fast in the same way. We should seek God, ask His direction and then follow the impulses we sense coming from Him. Some persons may be urged to fast on bread and water (the "best" fast according to Mary), others may be called to give up smoking, alcohol, or television. Others may follow the former Lenten practice of eating two small meals not to exceed the third meal. Fasting is not always "not eating." Some may do penance by eating what they don't like, or not speaking the sharp remark to a fellow worker or friend. Whatever we are called upon to do, we ought to fast with the same vigor and enthusiasm as we respond to Mary's call to deeper prayer. The important dimension is that we **begin to fast** and to allow God to use the fasting to move us forward on our way of holiness. As we go deeper and deeper into the path God has laid out for us, we will also change our way of fasting, ultimately, perhaps, reaching the "best fast," as explained by the Mother of God.

During Lent, 1988, Mary reportedly told the pilgrims gathered on Mt. Podbrdo that she was pleased with their fast and their Lenten penances, but she would be more pleased if they would fast from sin. Mary is our Mother, our model, and our teacher. Through the messages at Medugorje, Mary is educating us along the way of holiness and inviting us to be converted to her Son, Jesus Christ. Mother that she is, she desires each of us to become holy and to grow in God's love. Fasting is an important dimension in this growth.

Let us begin by asking Mary to intercede for us so that our minds will be open to hear the message proclaimed here and that our hearts will be changed to follow Mary's call to fast.

Sister Isabel Bettwy
Editor

8

INTRODUCTION

My purpose in writing this booklet is to encourage you to fast. At the end of this booklet, I would like to say to you, "Begin to fast," and I hope you will respond, "I will." I pray that, through fasting you will discover all the treasures that God has put inside you and that through fasting your longing for God will grow within you from day to day. I pray that through fasting you will discover the God of love, of hope, of faith, and of peace; and that through fasting you will also meet fellow travelers, and you will meet them in love, in peace, in trust and in hope. Through fasting, you will receive the strength to overcome the evil that is within you, because fasting should serve that cause also. And so, as we begin, may Almighty God bless you through Mary, the Queen of Peace, the Father, the Son and the Holy Spirit. Amen.

FASTING IS NECESSARY

Time and time again, the evangelists speak about fasting and report that Jesus recommended fasting to make progress in the spiritual life. What Jesus has said about fasting can be summed up in this way:

— Fasting is as necessary as prayer (cf. Mt 6:16).

— The resolution to fast (or to pray) ought to be a pure intention, free from all self-righteousness or pride. Consider the case of the Pharisee who used His prayer to show off his piety and to express his contempt for the publican, a truly humble man (cf. Lk 18:9-14).

— Jesus declared that His disciples would fast just like John's disciples, but not until He would have departed from this world: "As long as the bride-groom is present, the wedding guests do not fast" (cf. Mt 9:15-16).

— When Jesus explained to His disciples why they were unable to deliver a man from demonic possession, He ascribed a special power to fasting. On that occasion He stated that certain demons cannot be expelled except by prayer, and the evangelist Mark adds, ". . . and by fasting" (cf. Mk 9:29).

— According to Luke, Jesus did not eat for the forty days He was in the desert. In other words, Jesus fasted before proclaiming the Gospel. This was immediately after His baptism in the river Jordan (cf. Lk 4:1-4). While Jesus did not explicitly command His disciples to practice fasting, it would seem obvious that He expected them to do so.

FASTING IN THE EARLY CHURCH

Fasting formed part of the Jewish tradition, and it is known to have been practiced also in Greco-Roman civilization. The Jewish tradition recommended only one official fast-day, the Day of Atonement, which was a day of devotion. However, people would often fast twice a week, on Monday and on Thursday (cf. Lk 18:22). From the Old Testament we learn that at the time of great difficulties kings and prophets would ask the people to fast and to pray (cf. Jon 3:7). In the Psalms we find revealing verses, such as, "When they were sick, I put sackcloth on, I humbled my soul with fasting, murmuring prayers to my own breast" (Ps 35:13), or: "My knees totter from my fasting, and my flesh is wasted of its substance" (Ps 109:24).

The early Church introduced two fast-days a week, Wednesday and Friday. Some of the faithful would fast on Saturday as well, in preparation for the Lord's Day. The practice of fasting gradually became more and more widespread. A fast began to be kept for entire weeks, during Holy Week, for example; and as early as the third century, the Church introduced the forty-day fasting period of Lent, in preparation for Easter, the celebration of the Resurrection of Jesus.

FASTING REMAINS NECESSARY AS A SIGN OF OUR EXPECTATION

From a theological point of view, fasting would no longer be necessary after the coming of Christ, for the wedding guests do not have any reason to fast as long as the bridegroom is with them (cf. Mt 9:15). But since Jesus is still to return in His glory, fasting remains necessary as a sign of our expectation. That perspective gives new sense and meaning to fasting and since it makes us focus on the Lord who is to come, it now acquires an eschatological dimension.

In a word, we may conclude that the Church recognizes fasting, has been practicing it throughout its history, and has given fasting its true meaning. In certain religious communities fasting has been maintained as a practice up to the present day. By reading the lives of the Saints, we can ascertain that they attributed great importance to fasting. In the Rules for his Community, Saint Francis of Assisi urged his friars to keep three forty-day fasts during the year (Lent, before the feast of Saint Michael, and from All Saints until Christmas), and to fast every Friday as well.

Nowadays, the requirements of the Church are less strict. There are, in fact, only two days left when fasting is obligatory, Ash Wednesday and Good Friday.

Even before the events in Medugorje, which have restored fasting to the Universal Church, the practice of it went well beyond the minimum requirements of the Church among our people, especially in Hercegovina. This is undoubtedly due to the influence of Franciscan spirituality. There are many faithful, especially among the young girls and the mothers of families, who fast on Tuesday (Saint Anthony's day), for the twelve days before the feast of the Assumption, on the vigil of great feastdays, and during Lent. There was a time when our people (from Medugorje and the surrounding areas) would keep a strict fast even in the summer, during the heavy work in the fields.

A NEW REVIVAL OF ITS PRACTICE

The so-called "messages," like any of the other elements that lend authenticity to an apparition, cannot contain new revelations about God's plans concerning us, nor can they reveal new truths regarding the Church. Such "messages" could not possibly innovate or modify the revelation given by Jesus to the Apostles. Apparitions are always a sign that God continues to address Himself to

His children, and to encourage us to persevere on our journey towards Him. Most often He calls us through the mediation of Mary. Sometimes Jesus Himself speaks to us. Such interventions are no more than an encouragement to keep up practices that have been known and have been traditional for a long time. The call to fasting at Medugorje which Mary directs to our age is only a repetition of what Jesus had already said, and of what the early Church had put into practice and with such great zeal.

When we study the Old Testament, and examine in detail the various situations in which the people were urged to fast in those days, we find that prayer and fasting could bring about change or relief even in the most critical situations.

OUR LADY WANTS
TO REEDUCATE US

Let us now look at fasting in the context of our own time. When Our Lady asks us to say the Apostles Creed every day, it would seem that she wants to show us, in this way, that we live in an "impious" situation. She certainly wants to tell us something like this: "It is not enough to say the Creed; one must radically adhere to God who has given himself to us in an ineffable way in the person of Jesus Christ." That is Our Lady's method of giving instruction. It is interesting to note that, like all good teachers, she assigns concrete tasks.

Her request that we fast is in accordance with the tradition of the Church. We can also go on record as saying that her view of our age - which is almost exclusively interested in money, profit, the accumulation of material wealth, greed, and so on—is correct. Our Lady wants to re-educate us. But where should she begin?

FASTING WILL LEAD US TO A NEW FREEDOM OF HEART AND MIND

In the first place, Mary calls upon us to pray and to fast. By prayer we attach ourselves to God and by fasting we detach our heart from the good things that tie us to the affairs of this world. **Fasting will lead us to a new freedom of heart and mind**. Fasting is a call for conversion directed to our body. In a word, it is the process by which we become free from and independent of all material things. And as we free ourselves from things outside of ourselves, we also free ourselves from the passions within us that are keeping our interior life in chains. This new freedom will make room in our body for new values. Therefore, fasting liberates us from a certain bondage and sets us free to enjoy happiness.

AN ACTUAL EXPERIENCE

To confirm what I have said so far, I quote a testimony just as it was given to me by a pilgrim to Medugorje.

"I had begun to fast because my wife and my children did it; I did not want my wife to cook for me alone. At first, nothing remarkable happened. I knew that I was distracted in my prayers. I would listen to the word of God, but I did not experience any noticeable effect from it and did not have the impression that I was changing under its influence. I would listen to it and then go about my business, but nothing in me was changed.

One day it became imperative to me that I change my manner of praying. It seemed to me that my new view of prayer was the result of the silent reflection which was brought about during my days of fasting. In the beginning I was constantly battling my need to eat and drink, and would then put off my prayer till the following morning. Once, something happened which clearly demonstrated the efficacy of prayer. For a long time I had been on bad terms with my brother, and I had grown accustomed to that situation. We were not on speaking terms, and it did not bother me in the least that our wives and children did not know each other at all. Approximately one year after I had begun to fast, I became aware that the situation was causing me distress and making me uneasy. I continued to pray and fast. And then, one morning, I had the extraordinary feeling of being relieved of a burden. I went to see my brother and asked his forgiveness. He was ready also. Praise the Lord, and thanks be to Him! Now we live as true brothers. Right now, that is the most important thing to me."

WHAT IS NEEDED IS A RADICAL RETURN TO GOD

Reading this testimony, we notice that fasting was a help to this man in finding his own self again and in having another close look at his relation to God and to other people. As soon as his prayer began to bear fruit in his heart, he did not have to wait long for his new relatioship with God to flow over into a renewed relationship with his brother. How well this example proves that the evil acts of man cause him blindness! What is needed to make the disposition of our heart and mind change is a resolute, radical return to God. Fasting facilitates this return.

Fasting is not an end in itself, but it serves towards conversion: first, on the level of faith, and then, on the social level.

FASTING ASSURES US OF
A DYNAMIC STRENGTH

A radical return to God is impossible without prayer. Prayer will increase in quality and become free when it is combined with fasting. If we are convinced that the Virgin Mary asks each one of us to be her "mouthpiece" in this atheistic world, we ought to be willing to fast, and this fasting will then assure us of a dynamic strength.

When we begin to think of ourselves as the masters of life and of the world, and begin to behave accordingly, as if we had no need of God, we show the premonitory signs of atheism. Fasting is the best means to detect such predispositions in our heart. Fasting helps us to cling to the will of God, to understand it better, and thereby, to understand ourselves better. In speaking about fasting, L. Rupcic has said: "The reason and the primary value of **fasting is to be at the service of the faith**. It is a simple means which allows man to show, to strengthen, and to stabilize his self-control. Fasting is the guarantee of his surrender to God in true and sincere faith. As long as man is not yet master of himself (of his senses), he will be unable to place himself completely in the hands of God."

We know that in the Scriptures, Jesus tells us to pray without stopping, without ceasing. But on the other hand, day after day we find excuses, and we say we have no time to pray, or we say that the rhythm of our life is such that we cannot pray. But the depth of the problem does not lie in whether we have time or do not have time for prayer. Rather, the problem is whether we know the longing or the necessity for God, for meeting God through prayer. The more we have and the more we want to have, the less space we have for God and the less time we have for prayer. Or, at least we are in danger of not having space and time. In this way, we turn more and more to being practical atheists. That means, we are content to possess more and more material things, to have better food and better drinks, and we believe we can solve all our problems in this way. This way of behavior and these convictions exclude the possibility and the necessity of prayer.

Fasting has the special consequence of putting things into proper perspective. As a result of fasting we learn truths about ourselves more and more. We experience the truth of all things in new ways. Slowly and surely we realize more and more that we are not self-sufficient, and we realize that the whole world cannot satisfy the deepest needs of our human heart. Thus, a new way is being opened up for the conviction that we humans need God. The first Beatitude; "Happy are those who are poor in spirit, to them belongs the Kingdom of God," can be translated in another way; "Happy are those who have a desire, a longing for God." The person who is convinced that he is self-sufficient, that he needs nothing deeper or nothing higher than himself — that person is not poor before God. It means that he is living in the convictions that he does not need God, and there lies the problem of prayer. But slowly, through fasting and while we fast, this conviction bursts and we become more and more open for prayer, and that means we become more open for our meeting, our encounter with God. For that reason we can say fasting is something that cannot be replaced, but rather is something we definitely need. We need fasting to be able to grow in prayer and especially to grow in prayer of the heart. To say it succinctly, we find it easier to pray when we fast and we fast better when we pray.

There is an old proverb which states: "A full stomach doesn't like to study." The meaning of this proverb would not be altered if we changed it to, "A full stomach does not like to pray." The physical emptiness brought on by fasting helps us to realize our spiritual emptiness and need. The experience of a longing or deep desire for God does not go against the dignity of the human being, but rather, this longing confirms our dignity. We come to know and to experience our dependency on God and not on material things. This dependency on God does not turn us into slaves, but rather makes us free.

We are created for God, and God is always present for us. In the moment when we are together as friends, as partners for a contract, we feel good. If the heart becomes poor in the sense that it recognizes its need for God's friendship, then it will be more able to hear God's word in general. It will be more ready to meet people and put into practice this bond of friendship. That is the way to happiness. It is not happiness in the superficial, easy sense, but it is happiness in the sense of inner peace through which the person can be victorius in every difficult or unpleasant situation.

THROUGH FASTING OUR
HEART BECOMES PURE

It is now important to reflect upon another consequence of fasting. Through fasting, our hearts become more pure. We see reality in a better way. We find it easier to see what we have, what we need, and what we don't need.•We become free from the inner pressure of wanting and needing to have more and at the same time forgetting what we have already. Everything is relative in life. That means, things are not as important as we think sometimes. We live in a situation of believing that material things are very important. We forget the dimension of being pilgrims in this world. There are many people who would be happy if they had a roof over their heads and just a little bit of bread every day. And how much happier would they be if they had as much as we have. And yet, we often are unhappy and not content, although we have so much. The reason for the discontent lies in the fact that we don't see the essential anymore. We have become blind to the essential. Therefore, we are convinced that we need to have many things. With fasting, we find it easier to see the essential things of life. Therefore, fasting is so important. In making us interiorly free, fasting makes it easier for us to move towards God and towards people. In such a liberated encounter, reconciliation happens. The more we "meet" other people, the less time we will find for conflicts, negative things and wars. All conflicts happen because we are stuck to something.

•Many Christians are nailed to this world and cannot move. Through fasting they do not become pilgrims, but people on a pilgrimage who search for God and need God. That is the way to a new freedom.

Many people live in a situation of destruction, losing a lot of time and money on very unessential things. They cannot reach out and get through to the essentials. The pilgrim who is searching for God cannot allow anything like this to happen to himself or herself. Mary wants us, through fasting and prayer, to become real people searching for God, together with her. To become a pilgrim of this sort does not mean losing what we have, but rather it means developing a new relationship by being pilgrim people everyday, by being on a pilgrimage.

We are reminded of the Gospel parables where Jesus underlined the dimension of being on a pilgrimage. People who are on the road, on their way, don't allow anything to stop them. They are motivated and carried on by an inner hope of meeting the Lord. When people have lost that hope they begin to drink, to eat, and even to hit one another. In the Gospel of Matthew we read about the property owner who planted a vineyard, leased it out to tenant farmers and then went on a journey. When vintage time arrived, he dispatched his slaves to the tenants to obtain his share of the grapes. The tenants responded by seizing the slaves, beating one and killing another. We are also familiar with the parable of the virgins who had no oil. In these parables we see situations where the dimension of waiting was lost. In other words, Mary wants to make us always ready to move. She wants to guide us in growing in the knowledge of the essential and the unessential. Our hearts will become more open to those who are in need. We will find it easier to recognize the spiritual and the material needs of the brother or sister next to us. We could, therefore, speak about the social dimension of fasting.

Many people, in the beginning of the apparitions, asked themselves, "Why does the Lady not insist on social help and so on?" I believe she wanted to educate us for it before inviting us to do it. Over the years, many invitations have gone out and have fallen on deaf ears, because we are selfish and proud and we do not see the needs of others.

WHY FAST
ON BREAD AND WATER?

In Medugorje, the Madonna has asked for a
return to fasting. In response to the question,
"What is the best kind of fast?", the Virgin
responded, "Bread and water, of course." We
recognize that bread and water is not the only way
to fast, but it is the "best" way, according to the
Madonna. One has to grow into "bread and water"
fasting. If one has never fasted at all, it may be very
discouraging to begin to fast on bread and water
only, unless one receives a call from the Lord.
There are other ways of fasting which will
accomplish the same objectives in us and, at the
same time, help us to move toward the best fast.
For example, self denial from certain foods, eating
foods without seasoning, eating foods we dislike,
skipping desserts, and simply eating considerably
less at each meal are just a few ways of fasting
related to food. The important thing is that we
begin to fast in some way — now. In Medugorje,
however, there is an emphasis on fasting on bread
and water, and there is a profound meaning to it.

Bread is the food of the poor. To have or not to have bread is one of the essential questions of our existence.

The Bible often speaks of bread. God provided bread (manna) for His people during their journey across the desert (cf. Ex 16). In His teachings, Jesus speaks of the bread that has come down from heaven. An angel brought bread and a jar of water to the prophet Elija when he was exhausted from fatigue (cf. 1 Kings 19), and after eating and drinking, Elija regained his strength and continued his journey.

Is it not remarkable, on the other hand, that, according to the Gospel, the poor are closest to Jesus? They ate with him and followed Him and listened to His words. After speaking to a crowd, hungry not only for His words but also for bodily nourishment, Jesus multiplied the loaves (cf. Mk 8:1-9; Mt 15:32-39). By multiplying earthly bread, Jesus prepared the people for the Bread from Heaven.

The willingness to live on water and bread for one day shows a willingness to be poor before God, well-disposed towards His will. It means following in the footsteps of the prophets and in the footsteps of those who have been put to the test in order to give testimony to their faith.

Bread is the basic food of His people and at the same time bread is the symbol of life. Water is also irreplaceable in our life. Water is also a sign of spiritual purification. In these two truths the message is expressed: come back to life and live. Come out of your impurities and be pure. We are invited to live on bread and water two days a week. As the Madonna said, bread and water are the ideal fasting. The person who lives in this way, two days a week, is certainly doing something good to his body, spirit and soul. The Mother of God has invited us in full freedom. And so, that means that if we are very tired, or we have worked hard, or we are not in very good health, we must not be afraid to take tea or coffee and eat some little thing.

FASTING ON BREAD AND ON THE EUCHARIST

All that Jesus said and did concerning bread was aimed at the preparation of His audience for a new banquet, for the Bread from Heaven, in which He himself would be broken and shared for the redemption and salvation of mankind. In spite of all that Jesus did and said to make His contemporaries understand that His Body and His Blood were to be offered as food and drink beyond comparison, He was not understood. His audience rejected His message, pretending that it was a hard word and totally incomprehensible (cf. Jn 6:52, 60).

By choosing to eat nothing but bread on certain days, we can understand, by personal experience, what the real meaning of Jesus' message is. We have been given the possibility of finding out, through reason and heart, the total dimension of the message which Jesus has given us to consider, for it is He who stays present in the Bread. By being too attached to the contents of our plate, we run the risk of losing sight of our primary nourishment in which God offers Himself to us in a very special way. In order to become aware of the presence of that tiny particle of the Bread in our body, we must be willing to suffer physical hunger. Otherwise we risk contempt for the crumbs. If we give thought to the practice of the early Church, which our Orthodox brethren still follow today, namely that of the obligation to fast several hours before receiving Communion, we will more easily understand what was said above. If we fast thus for several days, the reality will become even clearer.

Perhaps the poor, who know the importance and the value of daily bread, have best realized the value of the Bread from Heaven. Many times, the heart of the rich has not been open to that "little" gift which conceals a gift of infinite value.

A lady from the parish confided to me that ever since she began to live on only water and bread every Friday, her Communion has been a more solemn event for her. She is amazed at the physical pleasure she experiences when she receives the Little Piece of Bread in Communion. Each time she is deeply moved, because she is immediately aware that through this Bread Jesus comes closer to her.

MARY'S MESSAGE ABOUT EUCHARIST

Fasting purifies our heart in order to open it wider to both God and people. Fasting makes us more receptive to the Word of God, and incites us to receive Communion.

New dimensions open up to us in the celebration of, or participation in Holy Mass and in the adoration of God and of Jesus in the Eucharist. The moment comes when the fact that we do not comprehend the mystery of the Eucharist is no longer important. What is important, however, is the fact that the Eucharist begins to come to life and to be active within us. In one message, the Madonna called all to "let Holy Mass be life for you." Then progress towards a new relationship, blessed with friendship between God and us, has begun.

THERE IS NO SUBSTITUTE FOR FASTING

To all Christians it must be clear that all persons who have been baptized, no matter what their social status or their position, are called to prayer. Nobody is exempt from this obligation, neither those in good health nor the sick, neither children nor people of old age, neither the learned nor the illiterate; no one is excused from prayer.

But not all are called to the same prayer. For example, a bedridden sick person has never been required to go to church in order to attend Mass; such a person has always been asked to say his prayers in bed. And, as far as children are concerned, they will never be required to pray like adults; they should be taught to pray in a manner that is fit for children.

The same is true with regard to fasting. We are all called to fast, adults as well as children, those in good health as well as the sick.*

• In the last few decades, fasting has been replaced gradually by works of charity. That we are all called to do good works is undeniable; it is one of the criteria by which we shall be judged at our death (cf. Mt 25:31-46).

*cf. The medical advice and the precautions to be observed in the practice of fasting are given by Professor Joyeux on the audio cassette **The Revival of Fasting Among Christians,** published by Editions Mambre, 23, Rue de Fleurus, 75006 Paris. It can also be obtained at Editions du Parvis, CH-1631 Hauteville/Switzerland.

It is also true that fasting is not part of those good works. Rather, good works are the fruit of prayer and fasting. They ought to be the expression of our self-denial and of our penance. Fasting has a greater and more profound significance, which deserves to be specified further.

To begin with, fasting and prayer combined have a common characteristic which can be very profound. They are both part of our Christian formation because they deepen our relationship with God and with our neighbor. For that reason, prayer and fasting are, in a way, two pillars of our faith-life.

Both the rich and the poor are called to fast. The poor must fast in order that they do not become totally embittered, for fasting will, in a certain sense, help them to free their heart from the burden of poverty. A poor man is not asked to give money to other poor people. His fast will allow him to accept his poverty and dignity, and thereby, to pull himself out of his condition more easily.

The rich should fast so that they will not withdraw within themselves. Because of their wealth, they run the risk of becoming alienated from their own nature, from their neighbor, and from God. Fasting will help them keep their priorities in proper order.

Fasting is one of the fundamental principles of Christian life; it makes the faithful capable of living in accordance with the will of God in all circumstances. Through fasting the will of God becomes more clearly recognizable and is less easily lost sight of. Just as breathing is the fundamental function of physical life in that it enables other functions to stay alive, so fasting and prayer are fundamental functions of the spiritual life.

FASTING AND PRAYER, A PROCESS OF PURIFICATION

Fasting does not require complete abstinence from food and drink. On the contrary, the messages state explicitly that on fast-days we must eat at least bread and drink water. In order that our fasting become easy and "sweet," we must pray much on such days. Prayer on fast-days is meant to serve as a landmark along the route we have to travel. From the very start, fasting delivers the body from negative forces; it allows the elimination of useless reserves and of surpluses that suffocate the body and weigh heavily upon it. Prayer protects us against the tensions and nervousness brought about by this process of elimination.

Fasting in itself does not make us anxious; but as the body becomes aware of the surplus suffocating it, the body begins to react. It is not uncommon (and understandably so) that a smoker who has begun to fast from smoking becomes aware of the shackles that tobacco puts on him. He would not have recognized this awareness otherwise. At the same time, the heart and mind become more inclined to seek an equilibrium between the forces of the spirit and those of the body, and to subject the body more and more to the spirit. This is always a very hard struggle, and prayer is a necessary help, therefore. For all these reasons, the Lenten liturgy sings that fasting lifts up the spirit and destroys vices. By strengthening his spirit, man becomes more resistant to psychological and physical illnesses. Thus, he lengthens his life since he is no longer weighed down by unused energy.

The numerous findings in Japan, in India, and especially in Tibet, confirm this. Only fasting can be the explanation for the attitude of the masters of spiritual life in those countries, who, by our Western standards, begin their spiritual activities rather late, often after they have reached the age of sixty.

By strengthening his spirit, man predisposes himself for free room in his heart, open to God and to neighbor. This is very important. In fact, if we do not have enough interior strength to forgive an insult, for example, or to forget an injustice, disastrous embitterment might encroach upon both our spirit and our body. In other words, fasting leads us to distinguish more easily between what is essential and what is not, and then we come to assume more readily an attitude that can cope with any situation. To the extent that our body is purified and freed from all constraint, our spirit is open to positive influences. It is well to note that our human nature is likewise exposed to "negative" influences, and that it is necessary to pray in order to counteract them.

We ought to see the prayer and fasting of Jesus in the desert in this light. It was in prayer and fasting that He entered into His conflict with Satan who attempted in vain to make Him turn away from the will of His Father. To the objection that Jesus' temptation occurred precisely because He fasted, we shall answer that it was through His fasting that He found the strength to overcome the temptation.

FASTING WITH THE HEART

In the messages from the Madonna at Medugorje we hear that we should fast with the heart. That is nothing more than what Jesus taught. Jesus judged those who prayed and fasted, and who thought they had the right to judge others because of their fasting and praying, but for whom the fasting did not bring about a changed heart.

In the first place, fasting with the heart means following the invitation to fast in confidence and trust even if we find it hard to fast. We should not lose confidence that God wants something good for us through fasting.

Fasting with the heart means that we should expect and accept the processes that begin through prayer and fasting, and we should embrace and carry them. We can expect our thoughts to change and we should look forward to growing in repentance and forgiveness. We should embrace the "pain" of fasting. Fasting with the heart means to accept fasting as a means of growing closer towards God and others. As long as we count all the things we have to renounce and we count the days on which we have to fast, then perhaps we are only on the way to fasting with the heart.

Fasting with the heart means loving and accepting our own way with God and with Mary. Fasting with the heart means loving freedom more than slavery to material things. Fasting with the heart means growing in love for God who is coming, and to whom our heart calls out everyday, longing for Him, as "the deer that yearns for living water."

Fasting with the heart also means deepening our joy in the Lord. For us it is enough to begin to fast with trust and to begin to go on the way of holiness. All the rest will then follow.

CONCLUSION

Fasting and prayer are not ends in themselves, but only means to recognize and to accept the will of God, and to solicit the grace of perseverance in carrying it out, in being open to God's plan, and in walking in the footsteps of Jesus Christ.

Along the same lines, fasting and prayer are the preeminently appropriate means to guide us in searching for peace. Those who are assiduous in their prayer and fasting will attain absolute confidence in God; they will obtain the gifts of reconciliation and forgiveness, and thus serve the cause of peace. For peace originates in our hearts and from there spreads to our neighbors and ultimately to the entire world.

Peace is something dynamic; it cannot be bought or sold. It prospers only in the hearts of people who are capable of forgiving and of loving those who have wronged and hurt them. Fasting is the prayer of the whole body; it is prayer through the body. Fasting shows that our body must participate in our prayer, and that our prayer must become carnal in order to be prayer in the fullest sense of the word.

In one of his books, Anselm Grun declares: "Fasting is the cry of our body which is seeking God, the cry of our innermost heart, our deepest deep, where, in our extreme powerlessness, we encounter our vulnerability and our nothingness, to throw ourselves totally into the abyss of God's incommensurability."*

Fasting and prayer do not concern us exclusively, even though they open up perspectives of new possibilities and new dimensions in our communion with God and with other people. God does not want to rob us of our time or to destroy us by our fast. On the contrary, He wants fasting and prayer to make us find our joy in Him and in our neighbor, so that we are able to live in union with

*Anselm Grun: Fasten, Munsterschwarzbach, 1984.

other people and thus to bring together in peace and love all the conditions that are necessary for our own happiness and that of mankind as a whole.

⁕The process is a difficult one; it is easier to give one's money to the poor than to forgive and reestablish good relations with our human brothers and sisters. Why not try to persevere in both? That is the only means of bringing about a return of inner peace which will then overflow into world peace — just what Our Lady has called for at Medugorje.

PRAYER ON FAST DAYS

On August 14, 1984, Our Lady said: "I would like the world to pray with me these days! As much as possible! To fast strictly on Wednesdays and Fridays; to pray every day at least the Rosary: the joyful, sorrowful and glorious mysteries. . ."

O Lord God, Creator of all creation and my Creator! Today I give you thanks for having arranged the world so wonderfully. Thank you for having given fertility to Mother Earth so that she bears us all kinds of fruit! Thank you for the food prepared from the fruits of the earth! Father, I rejoice in your creatures, I rejoice in all the fruits today, and I thank you! Thank you for our daily food and drink.

Father, thank you for having made my body in such a way as to be able to use the fruits of the earth and so develop and serve you. Thank you, Father, for all those who, through their work, produce new life possibililties. Thank you for those who have much and give away to others! Thank you for all who are hungry for Heavenly Bread while eating this earthly one! Father, thank you also for those who have nothing to eat today, for I am convinced that you will send them help through good people.

Father, today I decide to fast. In doing so, I do not despise your creatures, I do not renounce them, I only want to discover their value. I decide for fasting because your prophets used to fast, because Jesus Christ fasted and so did His apostles and disciples. I especially decide for fasting because your servant, Mother Mary, fasted, too. She called me to fast when she said: "Dear Children: Today, I invite you to start fasting with the heart. There are a lot of people who fast because others do so. Fasting is a habit nobody wants to give up. I ask the parish to fast out of gratitude that God allowed me to stay in this parish so long. Dear Children, fast and pray with the heart! Thank you for having responded to my call" (September 20, 1984).

Father, I present this day of fasting to you. Through fasting I want to listen to and live your Word more. I want, during this day, to learn to be turned more toward you, in spite of all the things that surround me. With this fast that I take upon myself freely, I pray to you for all who are hungry and who, because of their hunger, have become aggressive.

I present you this fast for PEACE in the world. Wars come because we are attached to material things and are ready to kill each other because of them. Father, I present to you this fast for all those who are totally tied down to material things so that they are unable to see any other values.

I ask you for all those who are in conflict because they have become blind in what they possess. Father, open our eyes, through fasting, to what you give us, to what we have!

I am sorry for the blindness which has taken hold of my senses so that I do not give thanks for the goods I have. I repent of every misuse of material goods because I used to judge their value wrongly. Make me able, through this fast today, to see you and the people around me better. Through today's fasting, let love for you and for my neighbor grow in me.

Father, I decide to fast today, (to live on bread and water) that I may better understand the value of Heavenly Bread, the presence of your Son in the Eucharist. Let my faith and trust grow through fasting.

Father, I decide for fasting and accept it because I know that in this way my longing for you will grow in me. Eagerly and with gratitude do I think of your Son's words: "How blest are the poor in spirit; the reign of God is theirs." Father, make me poor before you. Grant me grace that through fasting my desire for you may grow, that my heart may long for you as the deer for the running waters and the desert for the clouds of rain.

Father, I pray to you, grant that through this fast my understanding of the hungry and of the thirsty, of those who do not have enough of material goods, may especially grow! Help me see what I do not need, but possess, that I may give it up for the benefit of my brothers and sisters.

O Father, I especially pray to you, grant me the grace to become aware that I am but a pilgrim on this earth, that when passing away to the other world I shall not take anything but love and good deeds. Let the awareness grow within me that even when I possess something I cannot call it my own, for I only received it from you to manage it. Father, grant me grace that through fasting I may become humbler and more willing to do your will! So cleanse me of my selfishness and haughtiness.

Through this fast cleanse me of all bad habits and calm down my passions, and let your virtues increase in me. Let the depth of my soul open to your grace through this fast so that it may totally affect and cleanse me.

Help me to be always like your Son in trials and temptations, to resist every temptation, so as to be able to serve you and seek your word more and more, day after day.

Mary, you were free in your heart and bound to nothing except the Father's will. Obtain by prayer the grace of a joyful fast for me today, in which my heart will be able to sing with you a thanksgiving song. Obtain by prayer the grace for me that my decision to fast may be firm and lasting. And I offer, for all people, the difficulties and the hunger I am going to feel today. Mary, pray for me. Let every evil and Satan's temptation keep away from me today through your intercession and though the power of your protection. Teach me, Mary, to fast and to pray that day after day I may become more and more like you and your Son, Jesus Christ, in the Holy Spirit. Amen

Taken from:
PRAY WITH THE HEART!
Medugorje Manual of Prayer
By: Fr. Slavko Barbaric